MY FIRST BABY:

Anticipation and Preparation, Arrival and First Moments, New Parenthood: Navigating Challenges, Milestones and Moments of Wonder, Bonding and Building Connections, Sleepless Nights and Joyous Days, Learning Together:, Growth and Development, Support System: Family and Community, Reflections and Looking Ahead.

GIFTSON E. DAVIDSON

Copyright

TABLE OF CONTENTS

About the Author: Giftson E. Davidson

Giftson E. Davidson is a beacon of parental guidance, renowned for insightful writings that resonate deeply with new parents embarking on the life-altering journey of welcoming their first child. With a background in child psychology and a heartfelt dedication to nurturing familial bonds, Davidson's literary work has become a trusted companion to countless individuals traversing the maze of early parenthood.

In the book "My First Baby," Davidson delicately captures the myriad emotions, challenges, and joys that accompany the arrival of a newborn. Through poignant anecdotes, compassionate advice, and a wealth of practical tips, the author expertly navigates the uncharted waters of early parenting.

Each chapter is a testament to Davidson's profound understanding of the complexities of this transformative phase. From the anticipatory moments before birth to the tender first steps, "My First Baby" serves as a guiding beacon, offering reassurance and guidance to parents navigating the delicate terrain of nurturing a new life.

Davidson's empathetic approach shines through the pages, addressing common concerns, celebrating milestones, and fostering an understanding of the emotional intricacies inherent in raising a child. The book is a treasure trove of wisdom, providing not just information but also a comforting embrace for those navigating the uncertainties of parenthood.

"My First Baby" is a testament to Davidson's commitment to empowering parents, offering a roadmap through the beautiful yet challenging landscape of early childhood. With heartfelt prose and a wealth of knowledge, the book stands as a compassionate companion for anyone embarking on this remarkable journey of parenthood.

Introduction

The appearance of an infant proclaims a journey dissimilar to some others—the phenomenal section through the underlying year of life. From the moment their small fingers twist around yours to the provisional first steps, each achievement denotes a phenomenal development in a child's life. This fantastic journey through the first year is an embroidery woven with adoration, revelation, and development, a complex mosaic of minutes scratched in memory for eternity.

Following a child's appearance, time appears to transform into another aspect. Days are obscure, but every second is fastidiously carved in the heart. The underlying few weeks bring a fragile dance of adaptation for the two guardians and their infant. Restless evenings interweave with the wonder of looking into those honest eyes, eyes that appear to hold the insider facts of the universe.

The delicate hug of an infant, with their minuscule fingers folded over yours, connotes the beginning of a year-long symphony—an ensemble reverberating with laughs, cries, and the main babblings that pull at the heartstrings. Those early coos and jabbers structure the principal notes of correspondence, an unbelievable language that only a parent really fathoms.

As days transform into many weeks and months, the scene of change unfurls. Every month spreads out another section of revelation—turning over, getting to handle objects, the first tooth, and the continuous rise of their remarkable character. The fast speed of development is amazing, yet in the midst of the achievements, the pith of treasuring each temporary second remaining part is vital.

The child's most memorable year is an odyssey of 'firsts' —from the principal grin that lights up the space to the provisional initial steps that reverberate the victory of determination. Each achievement turns into a valued memory, a demonstration of the flexibility and marvel of life in its most flawless structure.

In the midst of the joyous minutes, there are difficulties that mesh into the fabric of life as a parent. The restless evenings and unknown regions of relieving a crying child test one's understanding, yet they produce a solid bond that rises above the domains of understanding.

A child's most memorable year isn't simply a time of development for the baby; it is also an extraordinary phase for the guardians. A stage uncovers qualities they never knew existed and brings out feelings that reclassify the importance of genuine love. The flexibility and versatility we saw during this stage are downright unprecedented.

The achievements accomplished in the primary year, both of all shapes and sizes, establish the groundwork for a long period of learning and investigation. They messenger the start of a delightful story, an account prearranged with adoration, nourishment, and perpetual miracle.

As the debut year draws near, it abandons an embroidery woven with minutes—minutes that embody the significant magnificence of seeing a day-to-day existence unfurl. A year engraves itself upon the spirit, making a permanent imprint—a year that embodies the sorcery of fresh starts.

The baby's first year is a timeless symphony of love, growth, and discovery—an extraordinary journey that etches its melody into the hearts of all who bear witness to its brilliance.

CHAPTER ONE

WELCOME TO PARENTHOOD

The baby's first year is a timeless symphony of love, growth, and discovery—an extraordinary journey that etches its melody into the hearts of all who bear witness to its brilliance.

Welcome to parenthood, an excursion that rises above the domains of affection, versatility, and limitless miracle—an extraordinary odyssey that reshapes the actual pith of being. The second a youngster graces your reality, a significant shift happens, spreading out an embroidery of feelings and encounters that shape the underpinning of an uncommon bond.

The beginning of parenthood is a combination of elation and fear, a hurricane of feelings that typifies the supernatural occurrence of life. From the moment you embrace your child, a flood of adoration immerses your spirit—an adoration so enormous that it knows no limits, rising above existence.

The excursion starts with the main shudder of life inside—a mystery divided among mother and youngster—an inconspicuous yet significant association that lays the foundation of this uncommon journey. Each passing second takes a stand concerning the phenomenal development from a small seed of life to a being overflowing with potential.

The appearance of an infant denotes the zenith of this journey, proclaiming restless evenings joined with delicate minutes—a sensitive harmony among wonder and fatigue. The delicate murmurs and little fingers getting a handle on your touch become the ensemble that coordinates the days and evenings of this new part.

Parenthood spreads out its layers, uncovering aspects of solidarity and strength already obscured. It's an excursion laden with difficulties—exploring the vulnerabilities, deciphering the subtleties of a child's cries, and figuring out how to flourish in the midst of the bedlam. However, inside these moves lies an inborn capacity to adjust, to calm, and to support—a demonstration of the unflinching soul of parenthood.

The physical and close-to-home changes are significant, both for the kid and the mother. From the thrill of seeing the principal grin to the tears shed during snapshots of vulnerability, every inclination turns into a brushstroke, painting the material of this common presence.

In the consecrated snapshots of isolation, in the midst of the cradle songs and 12 PM feedings, the transformation of a mother's personality unfolds. A change rises above the shallow, an excursion that cuts another character—one implanted with sympathy, strength, and a resolute obligation to support and safeguard.

The connection between a mother and her youngster blooms into a multifaceted dance of feelings—unqualified love entwined with a mystifying awareness of others' expectations. The simple demonstration of supporting your kid in your arms turns into a safe haven —a sanctuary of comfort and warmth in a world loaded with vulnerabilities.

As days transform into many weeks and months, the account of parenthood unfurls with its horde of achievements and esteemed minutes. The main chuckle, the provisional advances, and the murmured 'I love you's reverberation through the passageways of time scratched themselves as permanent engravings on the heart.

The emotionally supportive network encompassing a mother turns into the foundation of her solidarity. Whether it's the direction of experienced hands, the steadfast help of an accomplice, or the brotherhood of individual moms, these mainstays of solidarity give comfort during snapshots of uncertainty and cheer in wins shared.

Parenthood is a continuum—a steadily developing excursion that meshes itself into the texture of life's embroidery. It's a demonstration of the flexibility of the human soul, a depiction of affection in its most perfect structure—an adoration that knows no limits and stays unflinching through the preliminaries and wins of life.

In the midst of the endless penances and benevolent demonstrations, a mother finds a supply of solidarity—one that enables her to endure the hardships and lounge in the daylight of her kid's grin. An excursion shows the craft of equilibrium—sustaining the youngster as well as supporting oneself, for a sustained soul can all the more likely sustain another.

As the days unfurl into years, the reverberations of parenthood resound—a demonstration of the magnificence of sustaining, the strength in weakness, and the significant effect of unrestricted love. An excursion makes a permanent imprint—a tradition of adoration, versatility, and the sheer grandness of inviting a spirit into this world.

Welcome to parenthood—a journey that could only be described as epic, a tribute to cherish's perseverance through embrace, and a festival of the remarkable connection between a mother and her kid.

In the event that you thought there was a manual prior to having kids, you know, at this point, there isn't. Raising little individuals is an individual encounter, and I couldn't actually measure up to anything more. The affection you have for your kid, combined with the huge feeling of obligation of raising a genuinely living human, can surely push you to the brink of collapse, particularly when you're worn out, restless, and short on close-to-home assets.To start with, know this: You are doing a really respectable and astonishing thing by raising infants and little children, who will one day go out into the wide world and do something significant, stacked up with every one of the great things you showed them en route.

Every kid in your family will show you something new and call upon abilities you may, as of now, have or will foster over the long haul. Assuming you have more than one kid, you might find that every kid needs something else by and large. Answer the kid you have, not the one you read about in a nurturing book. Trust yourself to have an independent mind, to get to know your child and baby, and to learn and develop with them.Here are a few hints for those early, long stretches of nurturing, from somebody who has that old news and knows the number of blended feelings those early days can bring.

1.Be alright with not knowing all of the answers.

Feeling sure with nurturing comes in time and fluctuates as per what time of nurturing you are in. Those beginnings of nurturing accompany such a lot of data, when you are scarcely getting sufficient rest and everything can feel like a haze. Each phase of a child's or baby's life accompanies new inquiries and assumptions. Right when you feel like you're on top of everything, your little individual could arrive at another achievement or face another test, and it seems like you're once again at the starting point!Be good with following your stomach too, as a ton of nurturing counsel can clash with or conflict with your own qualities. Web-based entertainment, which is generally a social examination stage, causes every other person's feature reel to feel like evidence that you're missing the point entirely. In those minutes, the delight of this valuable honor of raising a family can be lost. Permit yourself a lot of opportunity to feel certain. Your certainty will develop with your experience.

2. Keep it genuine.Disregard Instagram's nurturing.

These depictions neglect to show the muddled minutes, and each parent has those. You are in an ideal situation, taking a rest, taking a walk, paying attention to music, observing some Netflix, or spending time with a companion or accomplice rather than losing all sense of direction in the correlation scroll. There are a lot of examinations arising that show the more time we spend via online entertainment, the more restless and overpowered we can turn into. Your child and baby need you to be okay. Try not to allow correlation to deny you that certainty.

3. Attitude.

Be kind to your mind. Our considerations accompany such automaticity, filling our heads with such countless messages, a significant number of them negative. Notice your opinion on your nurturing and your child and baby. Is it true or not that you are zeroing in on the thing you're doing adequately, or is your brain generally focused on what you wish you had done any other way? Might it be said that you are contemplating what you love about your child and baby, or would you say you are floating back to that not-insignificant rundown of things that are truly hard about raising a baby? At the point when the self-decisive contemplations come, recognize them, acknowledge their presence, and afterward attempt to consider something that goes against that. This makes for more adjusted contemplations, which can be precarious to accomplish in those early, long stretches of nurturing.Our mind's pessimism inclination implies we give immeasurably an excessive amount of consideration to our concerns and insufficient thoughtfulness regarding what's working out in a good way. Bring a second to record on paper or converse with somebody about pretty much everything you are nailing in nurturing—every one of the viewpoints you have high expectations about. Name how you're a decent parent and what you've been getting right. Then do likewise for your kid. It's not difficult to become involved with every one of the formatively tested ways of behaving and how we will determine them. This will normally sabotage our trust in ourselves and in our kids. (This doesn't mean you don't interview about what's hard or look for counsel from others.) This is just a way you don't remain caught in contemplating what's up and purposefully make space for seeing, which is common decency to enjoy.

4. Relinquish unreasonable assumptions.

I think a ton of the time it's not the nurturing itself that's debilitating; it's the steady shuffle of contending requests. Attempt to relinquish unreasonable assumptions about yourself. These could incorporate keeping things clean, staying aware of entirely nutritious dinners constantly, going to every one of the get-togethers you are welcome to, and going to classes and exercises you think your kid should enjoy. There is something to be said about JOMO (the delight of passing up a major opportunity). Figure out how to say 'no' assuming you're burnt out on saying 'OK,' and cut yourself some serious leeway.

Nurturing is a regular job that consumes the majority of your psychological burden. You really want your rest.

5. Parents as indicated by your qualities.

There are numerous substantial ways to raise a family. One of the main parts of doing this is knowing your qualities and passing them down to your children. This is best finished as a visual demonstration, where they gain from your being a living illustration of how to be in this world. Get to know your child and baby and meet them where they are, precisely for the individual they are. I recall when I was pregnant with our first of three youngsters. I had contemplated and worked with such countless youngsters and felt totally ready—until the genuine live child came into my life. I needed to toss out such a large amount of what I assumed I knew about nurturing, tune in with our delightful young lady, and figure out how to parent her our way as per our own qualities. (I additionally needed to discover that committing errors and feeling totally confused on certain days was extremely typical and normal.).

6. Figure out your disposition and character.

Youngsters are brought into the world with one-of-a-kind dispositions, character, and hereditary organizations. Understanding what to do when your most memorable conception has a mental implosion doesn't guarantee that you will find it so natural with a subsequent conception as well as the other way around. Try not to expect a lot from yourself. With regards to little individuals, regardless of how talented you are and how painstakingly arranged your routine may be, infants and babies frequently do whatever they might feel like doing, seeing the world for the most part according to their own viewpoint and answering it as indicated by their character, personality, and hereditary cosmetics. They can't resist. Conflicting results in your endeavors are not out of the ordinary for some time. Keep it together.

7. Acknowledge help.

Nobody can do this gig alone without gambling with wearout. Children and babies are so dependent on their folks for everything! You are one individual; there is no shortcoming in looking for help. People are an exquisite, compassionate species. As a rule, individuals are wired to feel elevated when they help other people. A significant number of us don't have family or companions to help, so ensure you are interfacing with your local area, neighborhood chamber, and libraries for child and little child occasions where you can associate with different guardians and your child and baby can be entertained for some time. Assuming your youngster is neurodivergent, this can be a lot harder. Associate with parent and expert gatherings that focus on neurodivergence. In my numerous years working here, these associations have been a lifesaver for families who can, in any case, feel disconnected and overpowered.

8. Figure out how to adapt to testing feelings.

You have heard it previously, I know; however, feelings truly are infectious. You get them from your kids, and they get them from you as well. It's simply normal to feel profound when you have a close-to-home kid before you. During childhood and toddlerhood, the surprises are, in many cases, more successive, so guardians can feel worn out, making it much harder to utilize adapting abilities and keep mentally collected. Simply continue learning and attempting. Children and babies are a lot more joyful when the adults in their lives know how to remain even-tempered in the tempest. Infants and babies (and youngsters and teens as well) utilize our condition of quiet to assist with quieting themselves. This is called a co-guideline. This is hard for the greater part of us, correct? Relax; a great many people I see about nurturing battle with this. Simply recall, at some point, one groundbreaking insight and each new conduct in turn, and we are a bit closer to fostering this expertise.

9. Apply empathy to your child and baby.

They are truly doing all that can be expected with what their bodies and brains are prepared to do, up until this point. They don't intend to intrude on your rest or espresso with a companion. I realize you know that. We as a whole know that, yet it can sure be baffling when you end up going for the stroll of disgrace out of a bistro when your little child has had an implosion on the grounds that the server served some unacceptable smiley face roll (who realize that the smiley face bread roll on the left had an additional spot on it).

These minutes can be overpowering and humiliating for guardians. Attempt and recall, children and babies wouldn't purposely humiliate their most loved individual on the planet (you). Their little creating cerebrum has recently closed down the reasoning part, leaving the inclination part on the cutting edge. They need love, time, and support to get back on course.

10. Apply self-sympathy.

You have just been nurturing for a short period of time. This is all new to you; don't anticipate knowing the responses without fail. Anticipate irregularities and vulnerability. This is everyday life, not an impeccably coordinated execution for public entertainment. At the point when you battle, don't be difficult on yourself. We, as a whole, battle. In the event that you have minutes and wish you hadn't, excuse yourself and, assuming you lashed out with your kid, apologize and be responsible.

11. Limits.

Last, yet in no way, shape, or form, put down certain boundaries and limits with your baby and more established kids. Babies and kids need our authority about what is and isn't satisfactory at home and out locally. They need to realize there are social standards to keep the social string durable. Youngsters need to foster responsibility through our sort, however firm limits. They will normally commit a lot of errors en route when their feelings and inner selves are huge. We must show empathy for this formative stage, sympathize with them about their sentiments, and afterward, put forth the line. Mercifully, let them know when their way of behaving is destructive to you or others. Assist them with gaining from it and improving things. Set them up whenever they are experiencing the same thing to be more managed and kinder. Assuming they mess up, don't address it; simply support them to improve sometime later and continue on. Babies and youngsters feel disgrace as well, so consistently show them your unrestricted love, pardon them, and outright take pleasure in them, even on the trickiest of days.

CHAPTER TWO

FEEDING YOUR BABY

Feeding your baby is an exquisite act that transcends mere nourishment—it's a profound connection, a symphony of bonding, and an opportunity to foster growth and well-being. From the very first moments of life, the journey of feeding intertwines with the essence of parenting, creating a nurturing environment that lays the groundwork for a healthy and thriving future.

The act of feeding a newborn is more than just providing sustenance; it's an intimate dance between caregiver and infant, a ritual that fosters closeness and builds an unspoken bond. As a parent, understanding the nuances of this journey—whether through breastfeeding or bottle-feeding—becomes a cornerstone of nurturing a child's development.

In this introductory exploration of feeding your baby, we'll delve into the multifaceted aspects of this nurturing act. From the intricate art of breastfeeding to the considerations and joys of bottle-feeding, this journey encapsulates the essence of providing not only nutrition but also comfort, security, and a foundation for healthy growth and development.

Join me as we navigate through the nuances, challenges, and joys of feeding your baby—an exploration that celebrates the profound connection forged through this act of care and nourishment.

1. EXCLUSIVE BREASTFEEDING

Exclusive breastfeeding implies taking care of your child's breast milk, as opposed to some other food varieties or fluids (counting baby formula or water), with the exception of drugs or nutrient and mineral enhancements.

Exclusive breastfeeding implies no other food or drink, not even water, aside from breast milk (counting milk communicated or from a wet attendant) for the initial half year of life, except for rehydration arrangements (ORS), drops, and syrups (nutrients, minerals, and medications).

Prédominant breastfeeding isn't equivalent to selective breastfeeding. Prédominant breastfeeding implies that the newborn child's prevalent source of nourishment has been breastmilk (including expressed milk or from a wet medical caretaker as the overwhelming wellspring of sustenance). Furthermore, the newborn child may likewise have gotten fluids (water, water-based drinks, or natural product juice), ceremonial liquids, ORS, drops, or syrups (nutrients, minerals, and medications). WHO and UNICEF suggest only breastfeeding babies for the first half year of life.

The ideal length of breastfeeding (WHO and UNICEF proposals)Start breastfeeding within 1 hour of birth.

Solely breastfeed your babies for the first year and a half of their lives to achieve ideal development, improvement, and wellbeing.

Unlimited exclusive breastfeeding brings about adequate milk production.

Assuming you are seriously sick or experience the ill effects of intricacies that keep you from really focusing on your newborn child or proceeding with direct breastfeeding, express milk to securely give breastmilk to your baby.

In the event that you are too unwell to even think about breastfeeding or express breastmilk, you ought to investigate the chance of relactation (restarting breastfeeding after a hole), wet nursing (another lady breastfeeding or really focusing on your kid), or utilizing donor human milk. Which way to deal with use will depend upon social setting, agreeableness to you, and administration accessibility.

It is workable for moms to breastfeed from birth only. In any case, a few ailments of the baby or the mother might legitimize suggesting that she doesn't breastfeed for a brief time or forever. These circumstances, which influence not many moms or newborn children, are recorded beneath, along with some ailments of the mother that, albeit serious, are not clinical explanations behind utilizing bosom milk substitutes. On the off chance that you are thinking about not breastfeeding or halting breastfeeding, the advantages of breastfeeding ought to be weighed against the dangers presented by the particular circumstances recorded.

Breast Milk might have longer-term medical advantages, like diminishing the risk of becoming overweight or large and creating noncommunicable illnesses like diabetes, cardiovascular sickness, and certain diseases, sometime down the road. Breastmilk shields babies from becoming ill and furthermore safeguards them all through their earliest stages and adolescence. It is especially successful against irresistible illnesses since it fortifies the invulnerable framework by straightforwardly moving antibodies from the mother. Breastfeeding is additionally a fundamental piece of the contraceptive cycle with significant ramifications for the wellbeing of moms.

Why Exclusive Breastfeeding?

• Exclusive breastfeeding implies that you give your child just breast milk — and that implies no water,food or recipe supplement.

• The American Academy of Pediatrics and numerous different specialists suggest restrictive breastfeeding until infants are a half year old.

• From that point onward, breastfeeding is prescribed for as long as a year, and longer as desired,while beginning on different food varieties.

• Just vitamin D drops are required for added sustenance — your child's Doctorwill give you a prescription

Exclusive breastfeeding is best for your child — better than giving your child both breast milk and formula. Infants who are only breastfed get the best medical advantages.

You can make it happen! Most moms can make sufficient milk for their children — adequately even for twins! At the point when you breastfeed only, your milk supply develops rapidly.

Exclusive breastfeeding is better for your child

• **Breast milk is extraordinary**. It has a novel mix of nutrients, different supplements and antibodies not tracked down in formula. Furthermore, unlike formula , breast milk changes as your child develops — so it gives precisely everything your child needs at each feed and over the long haul.

It even has a lot of water in it,so there is no requirement for different bottles.

• Children fed of just breast milk get less ear,stomach and lung diseases than infants given both formula and breast milk. Breastfed children are likewise more averse to foster asthma, particularly on the off chance that there is a family background of asthma.

• Breast milk is simpler to process than formula,resulting in less thrown up and obstruction.

Exclusive breastfeeding is better for you

• Breastfeeding solely assists rapidly develop your milk production. This will help you accomplish your breastfeeding objective all the more without any problem.

• It's generally all set! It's generally the right temperature, and there's no reason to wash and disinfect bottles.

• Since your child is probably going to be better, you will miss less time from work or school and have less visits to the specialist.

• Since your milk supply will be copious, you can keep on giving the advantages of

breast milk to your baby,through siphoning and storing your milk, when you return to work

Infants who have just breast milk for a half year become ill on rare occasions than children who eat different food varieties. They have less pneumonia and other respiratory diseases. They likewise have less digestive sickness, less ear diseases and less sensitivities.

Children are not prepared to take different food sources until half a year old.

For the initial half year of life, your child's digestive tract has little pores in it like a net. In the event that given different food sources, nonhuman proteins can go through the pores into your child's body and cause sensitivities. About a half year old enough, the pores in your child's digestive tract close up. Your child can then eat different food varieties.

Close to a half year old enough, your child can sit up. A child should have the option to appropriately sit up to swallow food.

Close to a half year old enough, your child's tongue can move in to acknowledge food, not at all like during breastfeeding when the tongue pushes out.

By a half year old enough, the child's mouth cavity has extended. Your child can then eat spoonfuls of food.

Breast milk ought to in any case be child's fundamental wellspring of sustenance for your child's most memorable year

Breast Milk is superior to some other nourishment for sustenance and infection insurance. It is critical to present solids following a half year so your child will figure out how to eat various food sources.

It's essential to breastfeed. Breastfeed before every dinner of solids, as the "principal course."

You can likewise keep up your child's bosom milk admission by continuously expanding feasts as they age. Attempt one feast of solids daily at half a year old, then, at that point, two strong feedings daily at 7 months old, three dinners per day at 8 months old, then three feasts in addition to snacks at 9 months old. Breastfeed before every feast, and when rest periods.

Significant fats found exclusively in breast milk assemble the mind, eyes and stomach related framework. The cerebrum and sensory system grow significantly over the principal little while. How much fat in your milk develops throughout this time. Breastfeeding through the subsequent year assists your child with fostering a superior mind, vision, and fostering a stomach related framework that all the more proficiently retains supplements.

Breastfeeding may go on longer than your newborn child's most memorable year of life Breastfeeding offers solace and daily reassurance. As your child fosters the capacity to talk and walk, the individual may likewise fear abandonment. Breastfeeding assists your child with having a good sense of reassurance.

As your child comes into contact with different kids, the infection battling parts of breast milk help that person stay solid.
The American Foundation of Pediatrics suggests restrictive breastfeeding for a considerable length of time, and proceeding to breastfeed as long as you both crave, even into the third year of life or longer. The more you breastfeed, the

more prominent the advantages, for yourself as well as your child.

You can breastfeed during pregnancy, as well as medical caretaker a more seasoned kid alongside a newborn child. This is called a couple nursing It even has a lot of water in it, so there is no requirement for different bottles.• Children fed just breast milk get less ear,stomach and lung diseases than infants given both formula and breastmilk. Breastfed children are likewise more averse to foster asthma, particularly on the off chance that there is a family background of asthma.

About a half year old, the pores in your child's digestive tract close up. Your child can then eat different food varieties. Close to a half year old enough, your child can sit up. A child should have the option to appropriately sit up to swallow food. When your child is close to a half year old, their tongue can move in to acknowledge food, not at all like during breastfeeding when the tongue pushes out.By a half year old enough, the child's mouth cavity has extended. Your child can then eat spoonfuls of food.

Breast milk ought to, in any case, be a child's fundamental wellspring of sustenance for your child's most memorable year.Breastmilk is superior to some other nourishment for sustenance and infection insurance. It is critical to present solids after a half year so your child will figure out how to eat various food sources.It's essential to breastfeed. Breastfeed before every dinner of solids, as the "principal course."You can likewise keep up your child's breast milk admission by continuously expanding feasts as they age. Attempt one feast of solids daily at a half year old, then, at that point, two strong feedings daily at 7 months old, three dinners per day at 8 months old, then three feasts in addition to snacks at 9 months old. Breastfeed before every feast and during rest periods. Significant fats found exclusively in breast milk assemble the mind, eyes, and stomach-related framework.

The cerebrum and sensory system grow significantly over the course of a little while. How much fat in your milk develops throughout this time. Breastfeeding through the subsequent year assists your child with fostering a superior mind and vision and a stomach-related framework that all the more proficiently retains supplements.Breastfeeding may go on longer than your newborn child's most memorable year of life.

Breastfeeding offers solace and daily reassurance. As your child fosters the capacity to talk and walk, the individual may likewise develop a fear of abandonment. Breastfeeding assists your child with having a good sense of reassurance. As your child comes into contact with different kids, the infection-battling parts of breast milk help that person stay solid. The American Foundation of Pediatrics suggests restrictive breastfeeding for a considerable length of time and proceeding to breastfeed as long as you both crave, even into the third year of life or longer. The more you breastfeed, the more prominent the advantages are for yourself as well as your child.You can breastfeed during pregnancy, as well as medical caretaker a more seasoned kid alongside a newborn child. This is called couple nursing.

EXPRESSING BREAST MILK

Expressing with a pump

Breast pumps are designed to emulate your child's sucking activity. There are two distinct types: electric and manual. With the manual, you just barely get the plunger and squeeze, while the electric accomplishes the work for you. Have a decent perusal of the guidelines and dive more deeply into your pump prior to utilizing it.

Ensure your pump and every one of the parts (bottles, valves, pipes, and so on) are spotless and sterile prior to utilizing them.

Assuming your child is in a medical clinic because they are sick or premature, your maternity specialist will help you clean and disinfect the equipment.

Manual breast pump

In the event that you're using a manual breast pump, it will take undeniably longer than if you're utilizing an electric pump. The beneficial thing about manual breast pumps is that they're less expensive, easy to use, lightweight, and quieter.

Here are a few hints on expressing with a manual pump:

Wash your hands thoroughly. Ensure your pump, the container, and the parts are spotless and sterile before use. Get settled and loose—ideally in a warm, calm room where you can unwind undisturbed.

Begin by rubbing your breasts for a couple of moments; this assists with the let-down reflex. It can assist with checking out a photograph of your child.

Place the breast shied or pipe over your areola, and gradually begin to siphon. It might take a couple of moments before your milk begins streaming.

Switch breasts when your milk begins slowing down. Then, at that point, trade back again, as you might find you have more milk to express. You might find that one breast delivers more milk than the other; this is ordinary.

Whenever you've purged the two breasts, remove the breast shields and put a lid (ensure it's screwed appropriately) on the jug. You can either refrigerate it straight away or leave it at room temperature for somewhere not later than 4 to 6 hours.

Wash and sanitize the pump and the other parts.

Electric breast pump

On the off chance that you're utilizing an electric breast pump, begin gradually with the suction on the most minimal setting. The advantage of utilizing an electric breast pump is that it accomplishes the work for you and takes less time than a manual breast pump.

Here are a few hints on expressing with an electric pump:

Clean up. Ensure the pump, container, and parts are perfect and sterile before use. Get settled and loose—ideally in a warm, calm room where you can unwind undisturbed.

Begin by rubbing your breasts for a couple of moments; this assists with the let-down reflex. It can assist with checking out a photograph of your child.

Place the breast shield or funnel over your areola, and switch the machine on. Begin with a slow speed—or one that you are comfortable with. It might take a couple of moments before your milk begins streaming, but when it does, you can speed up.

Switch breasts when your milk begins slowing down. Then, at that point, swap back again, as you might find you have more milk to express. You might find that one breast delivers more milk than the other; this is ordinary.

Whenever you've discharged the two breasts, remove the breast shield and put a cover on the jug. You can either refrigerate it straight away or leave it at room temperature for close to 4 to 6 hours.

Wash and disinfect the pump and parts.

FORMULA FEEDING

What is a formula?

Breast milk may be substituted with formula. It is created using a unique powdered milk. The majority of baby formula products include additional vitamins and minerals and are manufactured from cow's milk. The fat in the formula also comes from vegetable oils.

Your infant is given formula powder in a bottle along with cooled, boiled water. Additionally, a ready-to-drink formula is sold.

Your baby's development is supported throughout the first six months of life when you give them formula. They are also eligible to begin solid food feedings at six months of age.

Most baby formulas include protein derived from cow's milk.

Certain formula items include protein derived from rice or soybeans. Babies that have trouble digesting lactose or the protein found in cow's milk may use these specialty formulas. The use of specialty formulations should only be done under a doctor's supervision.

What distinguishes cow's milk from formula?
Cow's milk contains protein and salt, which babies under the age of a year old cannot adequately digest, so they shouldn't consume it as their primary beverage. It may also cause a low iron level in their blood.

After your baby is six months old, you may add small quantities of cow's milk to their meals.

What distinguishes breast milk from formula?

For the first six months of life, breast milk and formula are both full meals.

The presence of antibodies in breast milk helps shield your child from disease, which is one of the key distinctions between it and formula. The immune system of your newborn is not completely formed at birth.

Breast milk's natural composition automatically changes to meet your baby's demands. While the ingredients in formula milk don't change, as your child grows older, you may purchase several varieties.

Moreover, formula milk has more protein than breast milk.

Why would I give formula to my infant?

For a variety of reasons, formula may be the best choice for both you and your child. You could:

not be able to provide your infant with the necessary amount of breast milk.own a medical condition or take medicine that prevents you from nursing.not be with your child all the time; for example, if you are going back to work, you will not have the option to breastfeed.

Others, such as dads, transgender or non-binary parents, adoptive or foster parents, or kinship caregivers, have suffered from sexual abuse or another kind of trauma involving your breasts, which means that you have chosen to use formula for your child.Mixed feeding is an option if you want to breastfeed but are having trouble or don't make enough milk. When your infant receives mixed feeding, they will get both breast milk and formula.

What kinds of formulas are there?

The majority of baby formulas are created using dehydrated cow's milk and other nutrients, such as vitamins and minerals.

There are many methods used to produce that formula:

formulas made with milk, derived from cows' milkSoy-based formulas, which are derived from soybean specialty formulae, are manufactured from "predigested" cow's milk, meaning that the protein has been eliminated, decreased, or broken down. There are other formulations that are hypoallergenic.Long-chain polyunsaturated (LCP) acids, probiotics, prebiotics, and antioxidants are examples of additional substances. These, according to the formula's manufacturers, make it more resemble breast milk. Nevertheless, this does not imply that your infant's digestion of these substances will be identical to that of breast milk.Three varieties of baby formula are commonly available in Australia:

Starter formulas, also known as stage 1, are appropriate for infants up to six months of age

Follow-on or stage 2 formulas: they are meant for infants between the ages of six and twelve months and often include more iron. It is not necessary to switch to a follow-on recipe.

Specialty formulas: they are made specifically for newborns who have an allergy to milk or certain foods or who have digestive, malabsorption, or intestinal issues. A thickening is added to anti-reflux (AR) formulas to help maintain the milk in the baby's stomach and lessen the chance of reflux. The use of specialty formulations needs to be supervised by a medical expert. You may even choose a specialty formula based on your religion or culture.

Specialty infant formula is not cheap. To lower the expense of feeding your child, discuss obtaining a prescription with your physician or the baby's pediatrician.

Arrangement and hygiene tips

Only use bottles and feeding equipment that have been washed and sanitized.

Fill each container as needed. Assuming you actually do have to store formula, place it towards the rear of the ice chest, where the temperature is coldest.

If your child has not completed the formula in the bottle in 60 minutes, discard what is left. Formula and bottles become contaminated once the child has taken them. Try not to store remnants.

Assuming you're going out, transport the cooled, already-boiled water and formula powder independently. Mix the two not long prior to feeding. In any case, keep the prepared recipe cold in an 'esky' (cold capacity holder), child bottle pack, or cold sack.

Never warm a recipe in the microwave. This can make the milk heat unevenly and lead to burns. All things considered, warm up each bottle in a container of heated water. Bottle warmers are another protected choice. Adhere to the guidelines given.

Continuously make up the formula as per the guidelines on the tin. Assuming that the recipe is made excessively light, it can cause unfortunate development, and your child will be hungry. If it's too thick, it can prompt blockage, and your child could become overweight.

Tips to pick a child formula

If your child is sound, was conceived full-term, and is not breastfeeding, you ought to offer a cow's milk-based formula prior to attempting some other sort of recipe.

The cost of a recipe is certainly not an indication of its quality. Words like 'Unrivaled' or 'Gold' are utilized by formula companies to convince guardians to purchase their items. Pick what you can afford.

Take a look at the number of scoops of the recipe that are expected to make a feed. This will provide you with a smart idea of how long a tin of recipe might last.

Read the labels and ensure you're picking the right recipe for your child's age.

Take a look at how much protein the recipe contains. An excessive amount of protein can increase the risk of your child becoming overweight or hefty later in life.

Give your child a couple of days to become accustomed to another sort of formula. Try not to switch brands on numerous occasions.

Will infants be adversely affected by formula?

A few infants are delicate or hypersensitive to a cow's milk-based recipe. The protein in cow's milk could make your child have reactions.

Your health care provider could propose a hydrolyzed formula, all things considered. The hydrolyzed formula contains cow's milk protein that has been separated into smaller particles.

How can I tell when my child is hungry?

It very well may be difficult to tell when your child is hungry, or, on the other hand, assuming that there is something different making them fussy. In some cases, you won't realize without a doubt that your child is hungry until you offer a feed.

Babies typically cry when they are hungry. Setting the nipple of the container in their mouth will make them calm, and they will begin to suck.

Attempt to embrace your child as you would in the event that you were breastfeeding. Cuddle them, check their eyes, and post for their prompts or signals.

Your child will suck and swallow consistently. They might look as though they're focusing on feeding. Your child's hands could be held, and their entire body appears as though it's centered around sucking. As they top off, their hands and bodies become more relaxed.

Breastfed children manage their own milk intake. They suck when they're ravenous and quit sucking when they're full. In comparison, if you are using formula bottles, you have more control over how much milk they drink.

CHAPTER THREE

INTRODUCTION TO FAMILY MEAL

Babies ought to start eating the same meals as the rest of the household at age one. Around six months of age is a good time to start serving your baby modified versions of family meals. If you're eating roasted carrots for supper, for instance, shred them for your toddler and puree them for your infant.

Additionally, always put aside your baby's portion before adding sauce or flavor, regardless of what you're making. Having chicken, please? Put the cooked, unsalted chicken for your infant in a food processor with low-sodium broth, and process until the chicken is pureed. (Serve between one and two tablespoons.) If you're following the baby-led weaning method, use a fork to shred the cooked chicken, moisten it with a few drops of warm water or olive oil to keep it from drying up, and offer one to two teaspoons.Make mealtimes enjoyable. Parents often fear that their infant isn't eating enough. Additionally, some parents could unintentionally urge their young children to eat more.

However, this kind of "force feeding" only makes things tense and might lead to a baby's bad associations with food. A better course of action would be to let your infant decide when it's time for their next meal. Children, after all, have an innate system of hunger and fullness that enables them to eat when they are hungry and to quit when they are satisfied. (People are always learning from infants!). This implies that you may rely on your infant to control their food intake by just consuming what they need at the appropriate times.

Ultimately, it helps to approach infant and child feeding in this way: You are the one who decides what, when, and where to feed your child. Furthermore, it is your baby's responsibility to choose whether or not to eat and how much. This way of thinking may help relieve tension and strain during meals and foster a calm, happy atmosphere that will support your baby's development.

Accept the mess.

Do you instantly go for the closest damp wipe when you think about puree-covered faces, streaky plates, and dirty fingers? While it's normal to want to tidy up after yourself, it's beneficial for a baby's growth to let them become messy while eating. Assured. Making a mess while feeding provides beneficial sensory stimulation and helps infants get more used to and at ease with food.

Although it may be difficult, try not to wipe your baby's face all the time. and just accept their eagerness to try the items you provide! Regarding the duration of meals, remain flexible. When they finish feeding, babies may become rather fidgety and have limited attention spans. This explains why, as a meal comes to a conclusion, newborns may start flinging food and become fussier. Just be ready for a shorter mealtime, and remove your baby from their highchair as soon as they begin to show symptoms of fullness.

Talk to your infant while you're eating.

Here are some entertaining strategies to make sure your child enjoys mealtimes and feels like a member of the family:

Engage them in the discussion with the family.

Having a conversation at the dinner table is a great way for families to stay in touch and close. Furthermore, studies reveal that the conversation that occurs at family meals might really aid in your baby's language development. Aside from conversing, be sure to make plenty of eye contact and smiles with your kid when feeding to help create a happy atmosphere during mealtimes.

Give them cutlery.

Even though your baby may not be able to use a spoon until they are about 10 months old, it is always beneficial to introduce them to one early on. Additionally, providing cutlery during family meals keeps your infant entertained, aware, and active. This might perhaps give you a bit more time to consume your own meal!

Serve an open cup to your infant.

Your infant may practice holding a tiny open cup during family meals. When a baby is six months old, you may start giving them a little open cup with one to three ounces of water, formula, or breastmilk. Selecting a cup with handles can facilitate simple grasping, although a little cup without handles is also acceptable. (For advice on how to get your child interested in a cup,Remain composed in the face of varying eating times. Don't worry if your young child isn't eating at the same time as the family just yet! Include your infant in family meals, even if they aren't really hungry. By doing this, you're giving your sweetie another chance to connect with the family and discover more about what it means to enjoy meals.

Feed the infant in their chair.

It may be tempting to feed your child on your lap, but it's far preferable to use a highchair. Your infant learns that eating is only done while sitting, which is the safest posture to lower the danger of choking, when they are fed in a highchair. Make sure your highchair features a footrest for your baby's comfort and the finest possible experience. For the greatest chance of including your little child in the family dinner, move the highchair as close to the table as you can.

Is your child prepared to eat solid foods?

There is just one meal your infant needs: breast milk or formula. For the first six months after delivery, exclusive breastfeeding is advised by the American Academy of Pediatrics.

However, most infants are ready to start eating solid foods by the time they are 4 to 6 months old, as an addition to breast or formula feeding. Around this stage, newborns usually cease pushing food out of their mouths with their tongues and start to acquire the motor skills necessary to transfer solid food from the front to the rear of the mouth in preparation for swallowing. Look for further indicators that your kid is ready for solid meals in addition to age. As an illustration:

- Is your infant able to maintain an erect, stable head position?
- Can your infant sit with assistance?

- Is your child licking their hands or toys?

- Is your infant straining forward and opening his or her lips to indicate a hunger pang?

You may start adding supplements to your baby's liquid diet if the answers to these questions are affirmative and your baby's doctor concurs.

What to offer

Continue giving your infant up to 32 ounces of breast milk or formula each day.

Begin with a basic step. Serve dishes made with only one ingredient that are sugar- and salt-free. When introducing a new meal to your infant, wait three to five days to observe whether they respond with diarrhea, rash, or vomiting. You may then serve meals made with a single component in combination.

vital nutrients. Important nutrients to consider in the second half of your baby's first year are iron and zinc. Iron-fortified cereal and pureed meats are good sources of these nutrients.

Introducing cereals

The basics of baby cereal. Combine 4 tablespoons (60 milliliters) of breast milk or formula with 1 tablespoon of a baby cereal made of just one grain and enriched with iron. Serve it without using a bottle. Alternatively, after feeding them with a bottle or breast, have them sit up straight and serve them porridge with a little spoon once or twice a day. Serve one or two tablespoons at first. Once your infant is comfortable eating watery cereal, reduce the amount of liquid and progressively increase the portion sizes. Serve a selection of single-grain cereals, such as barley, oats, and rice. A newborn should not be given rice cereal alone because of the potential for arsenic exposure.

Include fruits and vegetables. Introduce pureed fruits and vegetables made with only one ingredient—neither sugar nor salt—gradually. Give yourself three to five days in between meals.

Present finger meals with excellent chops. Most infants can take tiny quantities of finger foods that have been finely diced by the time they are 8 to 10 months old. These meals include pasta, cheese, soft fruits and vegetables, well-cooked meat, baby crackers, and dry cereal. What happens if my child refuses to eat at first?

Since the flavor and texture of pureed meals are

unfamiliar to them, babies sometimes reject their initial doses. It is best not to push feedings if your infant resists. Retry after a week. Speak with your baby's healthcare physician if the issue persists to ensure that the resistance isn't an indication of a disease.

How about allergies to certain foods?

When introducing complementary meals to your infant, it's advisable to offer them items that may cause allergies. Foods that may cause allergies include:

- Tree nuts and peanuts
- Egg
- Products made from cow milk
- Wheat, Shellfish, and Crustaceans
- Fish Soy

There's no proof that introducing these foods later will help avoid food allergies. Actually, introducing foods containing peanuts to your infant at a young age may reduce the likelihood that they may become allergic to them.

Give your kid their first taste of a highly allergic meal at home rather than in a restaurant, and make sure they have an oral antihistamine on hand. This is particularly important if any of your relatives have a food allergy. If there's no response, progressively higher doses of the meal may be added.

Juice is okay.

Give your infant juice just when they turn one year old. A baby's diet doesn't need to include juice, and juice isn't as beneficial as whole fruit. Drinking too much juice might make you gain weight and cause diarrhea. Juice consumption all day long might cause dental decay.

If you give your infant juice, make sure it is only made of fruit, and don't give them more than four ounces each day.

CHAPTER FOUR

ALL ABOUT DIAPERS

A diaper, sometimes known as a nappy, is a kind of underwear that, by absorbing or storing waste products to keep them from soiling clothes or the surrounding area, enables the user to pee or defecate without the need for a toilet.

Did you know all there was to know about caring for your child when you became a mother? How can I put the infant to sleep? For diapering, where should one begin? How do you interpret cries? You're not alone if not. The majority of us don't.

Types of Diapers

Simple principles apply to both reusable and disposable diapers: Reusable cloth diapers are better for the environment since they can be used again to diaper a baby, unlike disposable diapers that are thrown away after use. (However, there is always discussion over how "green" cloth diapers are.)

When should I change my diaper?

As neonates, they urinate around twenty times a day. The good news is that you don't have to change your infant every single time because of those very absorbent polymers. That would be really laborious if you did. Basically, you'd be changing your infant all day long.

Nonetheless, throughout the day, you should change your infant every two to three hours. You may let your baby poop throughout the night, but as soon as they wake up, you should change their diaper since the acid in the poop might hurt their skin.

Dr. Sears advised on AskDrSears.com that "leaving a baby in a soiled diaper for a long period of time or not adequately cleaning them with wipes at every diaper change can harm their skin, which often causes an unpleasant rash." It could also leave patients more susceptible to bacterial and yeast invasion, which might lead to increased health problems and pain.

DIAPER SIZES

Weight and developmental stage of the infant are usually taken into account when determining the size of the diaper. Generally speaking, a baby weighing up to 10 pounds should wear a newborn diaper (first few weeks of life size 1), 8 to 14 pounds should wear a size 1 (2 to 4 months), 12 to 18 pounds should wear a size 2 (4 to 7 months), 16 to 28 pounds should wear a size 3 (7 to 12 months), 22 to 37 pounds should wear a size 4 (18 to 48 months), 27 pounds should wear a size 5, and 35 pounds or more should wear a size 6 (older than 4 years old).

These are some additional factors to take into account when selecting a diaper size since, of course, not all children will have weights that correspond to the months in the recommendations.

Is the waistline tight or loose? It's too tight if you insert your finger inside the waistband and tug till it feels constricting.
Is the baby's bum covered by the diaper? There will be leaking if it isn't covering your baby's

behind, and it won't function properly.

Is the baby's tummy getting red spots from the diaper chafing? Going up a size is indicated by chafing around the waist, groin, and hips.

Have the fastening tabs moved to the hips from their original location in the middle of the groin? In such a case, it's time to assess.

TOILET TRAINING

Five pointers to help your toddler potty train in a few days

First tip: Get your child ready.

Whatever your strategy, one of the most crucial parts of the process is getting your toddler emotionally, psychologically, and physically ready for this major change. When kids know and comprehend what is going to happen next, they flourish. Children are more likely to be ready and able to complete the toilet training process in a few days if we can educate them about the procedure and prepare them in advance for what to expect.

Here are a few suggestions for educating your kid:

Allow children to pretend to be potty trainers by using their stuffed animals and toys.

Read literature with a toilet theme.

Three to five days prior to the process's official commencement, make a paper chain and cut off one link every day until it is complete.

Allow them to choose new underwear and toiletries from the store.

2nd Tip: Get yourself ready.

We frequently hear about getting your child ready for potty training and how to prepare them, but what about YOU? Getting your home and yourself ready for potty training on a mental, emotional, and physical level is equally as vital.

Make sure your child is prepared for potty training before making the decision to go ahead and do it. Some 18-month-old toddlers are ready for the potty, while others might not be until they are 3 or 4 years old. An interest in using the potty, the capacity to follow instructions, the ability to detect when they need to go potty (they may crouch down, grip their diaper area, or hide), and the ability to stay dry for a few hours at a time are all indicators that a child is ready.

CHAPTER FIVE

SLEEP AND SLEEPLESSNESS

Infants' Sleep (2–12 Months)

What to anticipate

Babies often sleep for nine to twelve hours at night and take naps of two to five hours during the day. Infants snooze for two to four hours a day at two months of age, and for one or two hours at twelve months. Be prepared for things like sickness or schedule changes to interfere with your baby's sleep. Sleep disturbances may also be momentary due to developmental milestones like pushing oneself up to a standing position and beginning to crawl.

Most newborns can sleep through the night by the time they are six months old and no longer need to be fed at night. But 25–50% of people still wake up throughout the night. The most crucial thing to realize about newborns and nighttime waking is that they wake up four to six times on average. Infants that are capable of calming themselves back to sleep, or "self-soothers," wake up for a short while before falling back asleep. On the other hand, newborns who wake up their parents and need assistance going back to sleep are known as "signalers."

Many of these signalers struggle with self-soothing because they have formed incorrect connections with sleep onset. This is often the outcome of parents making it a practice to rock, hold, or put their infant into their own bed in order to aid in sleep. Babies may eventually come to depend on their parents for this type of assistance in falling asleep. While this may not be an issue at night, it could cause your infant to have trouble going back to sleep on her own.

Infant Safety Tips for Sleeping

Adhere to the ABCs of safe sleep: infants should never sleep in a crib by themselves, on their backs. Your infant should always sleep on his or her back, including during naps and nights.

Never put your infant to sleep on his stomach or side.

Your baby may remain in the sleep position he chooses once he can roll from his back to his stomach and from his stomach to his back. But put your kid to sleep on his back every single time.

Your infant should be placed in a safety-approved crib with slats no more than 2-3/8 inches apart, on a firm mattress.

During sleep, make sure your baby's head and face remain exposed and free of blankets and other covers. If a blanket is used, make sure your child is laid down in the crib "feet-to-foot," meaning with their feet at the bottom and the blanket tucked in around the mattress no higher than chest level. Take out every cushion in the crib.

Make an area that is "smoke-free" around your child.

Keep your baby's bedroom at a temperature that is appropriate for an average adult to prevent overheating while they sleep.

When your baby starts to pull up in the crib, at about five months old, remove any hanging toys and mobiles from the crib.

When your infant is around 12 months old and can start to climb, remove the crib bumpers.

It takes a lot of labor to care for a newborn, and you may not anticipate how often the tiny one will cry. When your infant screams, you should always comfort them. However, there are instances when you may not be able to stop sobbing, no matter how hard you try. Remember this if your kid isn't stopping screaming and you're feeling overwhelmed:

Your infant may cry a lot since this is how all babies communicate.

Around two weeks of age, babies begin to scream more regularly.

The second month of life is when crying grows and peaks, although it may continue until your baby is four to five months old.

Babies often scream more at night.

Tears might flow for as long as thirty to forty minutes. Even with healthy and typical newborns, they might cry for up to four or five hours per day.

Even though they may not be in pain, babies often scream uncontrollably when they are not.

It's OK to let your infant cry when they need to in order to release tension.

You can have periods of crying that you don't understand why.

No matter what you do, crying may not cease for a long time.

Eventually, the tears will end.

It's common for a baby to cry, and it's also common to get irritated when they refuse to stop. You may sometimes feel as if you are about to lose control at that very moment. Don't shake the infant at that precise time. You are a caretaker or parent, after all. Your stamina, tolerance, and patience are finite. It's common to experience feelings of helplessness, overwhelm, and even rage at a baby's incessant demands. Throwing, shaking, or putting the baby down roughly will never help, no matter how terrible things become or how exhausted and upset you are. Rather, soothe both yourself and your infant.

There will be an end to the sobbing.

Why do newborns scream so much?

Babies communicate via crying. While differentiating between a newborn's screams might be difficult, as newborns become bigger, parents can sometimes tell the difference between an "I'm hungry" cry and an "I'm tired" cry.

Infants weep because they are

- Hungry and uneasy
- Angry
- Weary and lonely

Cries may often be readily placated with food or a change of diapers. Never ignore your baby's screams. Picking up crying newborns is not a way to "spoil" them. When a newborn has no other means of expressing herself, being held is calming and comforting.

Even though newborns scream to communicate, they may cry for extended periods of time without showing any signs of what is wrong. Tears may come and go in an instant, leaving no trace behind. Your child is not attempting to make you seem like a horrible parent or to be angry with you.

How to soothe a screaming infant

- Prioritize your bodily needs.

- Is the infant dehydrated or hungry?

- Does the person need burping?

- How hot or chilly is it?

- Do they have soiled diapers?

After confirming that they are comfortable for the aforementioned tasks, look for any indications of a fever or sickness. Take the infant to the doctor right away if you suspect illness.

Is your child is in good health

If your baby isn't in need of anything physically, try one of these strategies to soothe your fussy child:

You may stroll beside the infant, rock them, or hold them close.

Get up, keep the infant near, and bend your knees many times.

Sing or converse in a calming tone with the infant.

Caress the infant's back, chest, or abdomen gently.

Attempt to divert the infant with a rattle or toy, or offer them a pacifier.

Cover the infant with a cozy blanket.

Put the infant in a car seat or stroller and go for a drive.

Play some music or activate some sound, like a clothes drier or vacuum sweeper.

Take a few minutes to try each of the aforementioned before moving on to anything else, or attempt a few at once.

If all else fails, feel free to leave the child in a secure location, such as a crib or infant seat, while you take some time to collect yourself. Get out of the room. Close the door behind you. Inhale deeply a few times. Give a friend or relative a call.

CHAPTER SIX

COLIC

Frequent, inexplicable weeping bouts that often last about three hours or more are known as infant colic. Although the exact reason is unclear, suggestions include dietary allergies, intestinal immaturity, and "wind" or "gas." Without medical intervention, colic usually goes away in a few weeks.

A baby with colic may not always have any health issues. Colic fades on its own with time.

How Can I Tell Whether My Tears Are Normal or Colic?

A unique pattern of sobbing is called colic. Although they are eating and developing normally, babies with colic scream sometimes.

At the same time of day, the spells are cast. The sobbing usually begins in the early evening.

When experiencing colic, a baby:

has difficulty calming high-pitched sobbing or shouting; may have pale skin around the lips or a crimson face; may tighten their fists, draw their knees in, or straighten their arms.

Could It Not Be Colic?

Other than colic, there are other reasons why babies cry. Making sure a baby has no medical reason to be crying is the first step.

Make an immediate call to your doctor if your baby:

- has a temperature of 100.4°F (38°C) or higher;
- is less awake or active than normal; isn't eating properly;

- isn't sucking vigorously when using a bottle or breast;

- has loose stools or blood in the stool;

- is throwing up (or spitting food out of their mouth or nose)

- not gaining weight or losing weight, and cannot, regardless of what you do, settle down.

Why Does Colic Occur?

It is unclear to doctors what causes colic. It could be the result of digestive issues, a baby's reaction to something in the formula, or something the nursing mother is consuming. Alternatively, it might be the result of a newborn attempting to acclimate to the sights and noises of the outside world.

Some infants who are colicky also have gas because they inhale so much air when they scream. However, the gas is not the reason for the colic.

Usually beginning between two and five weeks of age, colic usually clears itself by the time the infant is three to four months old. Colic may afflict any newborn.

How Is a Case of Colic Made?

For colic, there is no test. Medical professionals inquire about the infant's crying and general well-being. To be sure there's no medical explanation for the sobbing, they'll do an examination. Give your doctor a call if you suspect your baby has colic.

How Do They Treat Colic?

The condition known as colic cannot be cured. However, there are ways you may assist:

Verify that your infant is not starving.

Ensure that the diaper on your infant is clean.

During feedings, try burping your infant more often.

If your infant is being bottle-fed, experiment with different bottles to see if they reduce air swallowing.

Consult your physician to see if a different formula could be helpful.

Reducing their intake of caffeine, dairy, soy, eggs, almonds, and wheat may be beneficial for nursing mothers. Consult your physician before beginning this, and only discontinue one item at a time.

- Walk or rock the infant.

- Talk to or sing to your child.

- Give the infant its pacifier.

- Use a stroller to take the infant on a journey.

- Breathe slowly and calmly while keeping your infant nestled against your body.

- Take the infant for a warm bath.

- Rub or pat the infant's back.
soothing

- Lay your infant on your lap, stroke their back, and place them across your lap.

- Place your infant on a vibrating seat or swing. It might be a calming motion.

- Take your kid for a journey in the rear of the vehicle after placing them in an infant car seat. The car's motion is usually soothing.

- Play some music; sound and movement might help some infants relax.

Certain infants don't need as much stimulation. Babies less than two months old may do well in a crib, laying on their back, and with extremely dim or low lighting. Verify that the swaddle is not very tight. When the infant can turn over on its own, stop swaddling.

What Happens if a Baby Cries All the Time?
It might be difficult to care for a colicky infant. If your infant persists in crying:

Make a call to a friend or relative to offer assistance or to watch the child while you have a moment to yourself.

If all else fails, place the infant on his or her back in a crib devoid of plush animals or loose blankets, shut the door, and return after ten minutes to see how the child is doing. Do anything to attempt to de-stress and find some calmness during those ten minutes. Consider doing a face wash, having a snack, taking slow breaths, or enjoying some music.

Nobody is to blame for your baby's weeping when they have colic—neither you nor them. Remain calm and aware that your child will grow out of this stage.

Put the baby down in the crib and get assistance immediately if you ever feel like you might harm yourself or the child.

Conclusion

"In the tapestry of life, welcoming my first baby has woven a chapter of unparalleled significance. From the tender anticipation of their arrival to the sheer wonder of witnessing their first steps, this journey of parenthood has been an extraordinary revelation.

Each moment, from the sleepless nights to the heart-melting smiles, has etched itself upon the canvas of my heart, creating a masterpiece of love, growth, and endless discoveries. Navigating this uncharted terrain of nurturing a life has been a testament to resilience, patience, and boundless affection.

As I reflect on this transformative voyage, I am humbled by the sheer magnitude of love—a love that knows no bounds and continues to deepen with each passing day. The milestones achieved and the hurdles overcome have not only shaped my child's growth but have also sculpted my own evolution as a parent.

The support and guidance received from loved ones and the community have been invaluable—a reminder that this journey of parenthood is not walked alone. Together, we celebrate the victories, learn from the challenges, and cherish every moment that contributes to this intricate mosaic of parenthood.

As I gaze into the future, I am filled with anticipation—a sense of wonder at the adventures yet to unfold, the lessons waiting to be learned, and the myriad of memories waiting to be made. My first baby has bestowed upon me a gift beyond measure—a gift of immeasurable love and an unbreakable bond that transcends time.

This conclusion marks not an end but a continuation—a continuation of a lifelong journey of love, growth, and an everlasting connection forged in the beautiful tapestry of parenthood."